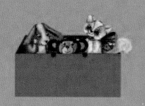
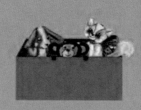

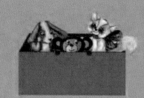
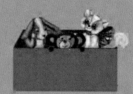

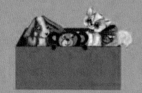
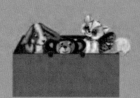
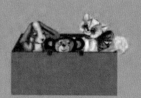

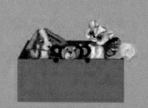
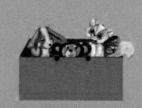

My Truly Most Favorite Fluffy Friend
Emma and Friends Book 3

I Do Not Like Bugs!

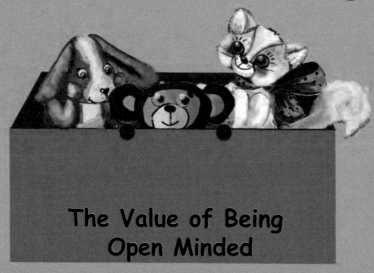

The Value of Being
Open Minded

Author: Pamela Tomlin

Illustrator: Tamara Piper

To Kayleigh, Jon, and Paul.
They each had a part in providing
inspiration for this story.

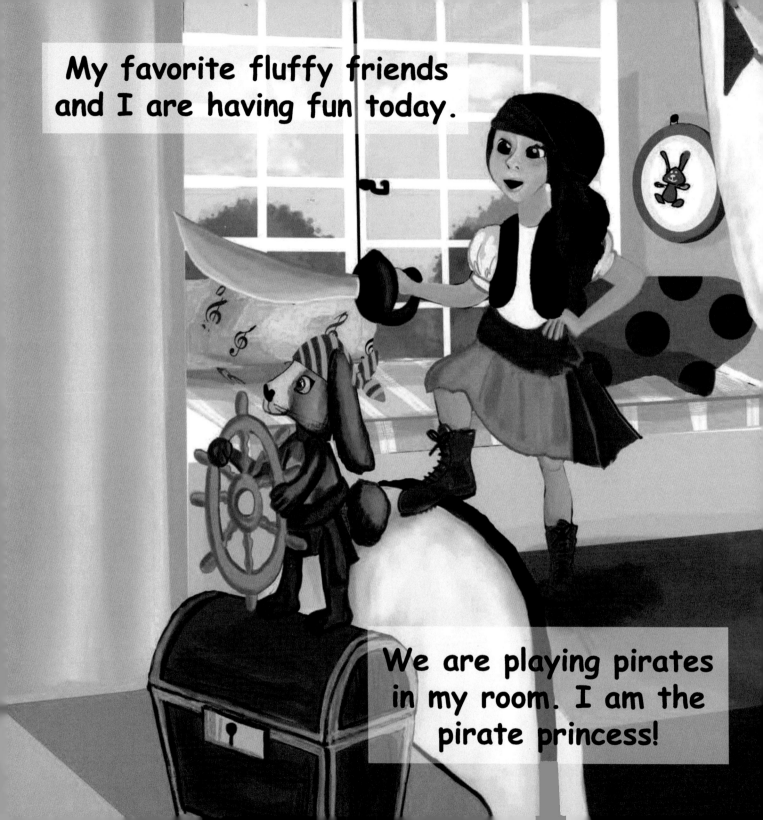

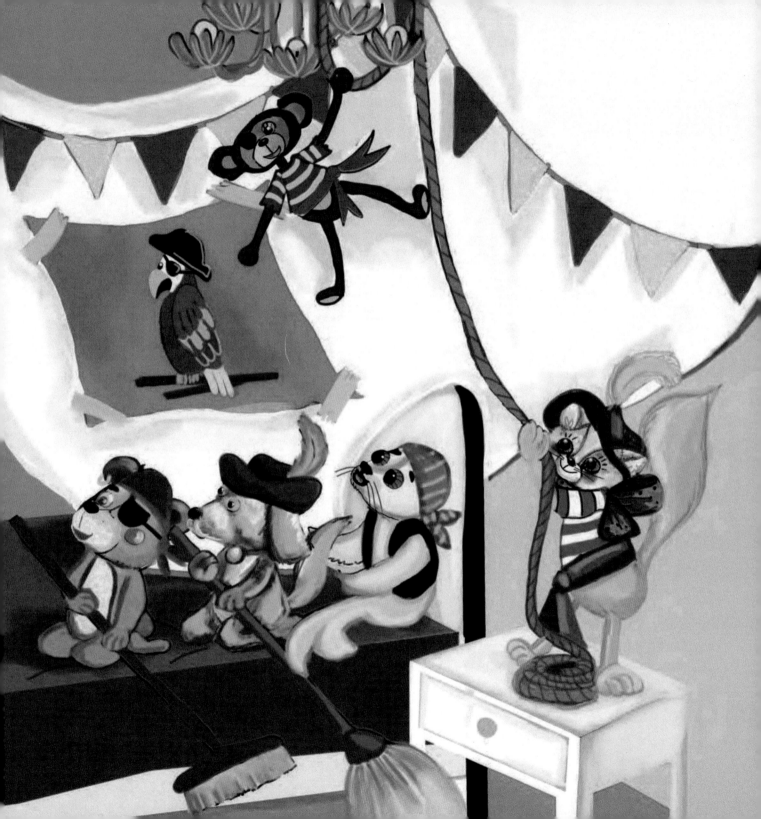

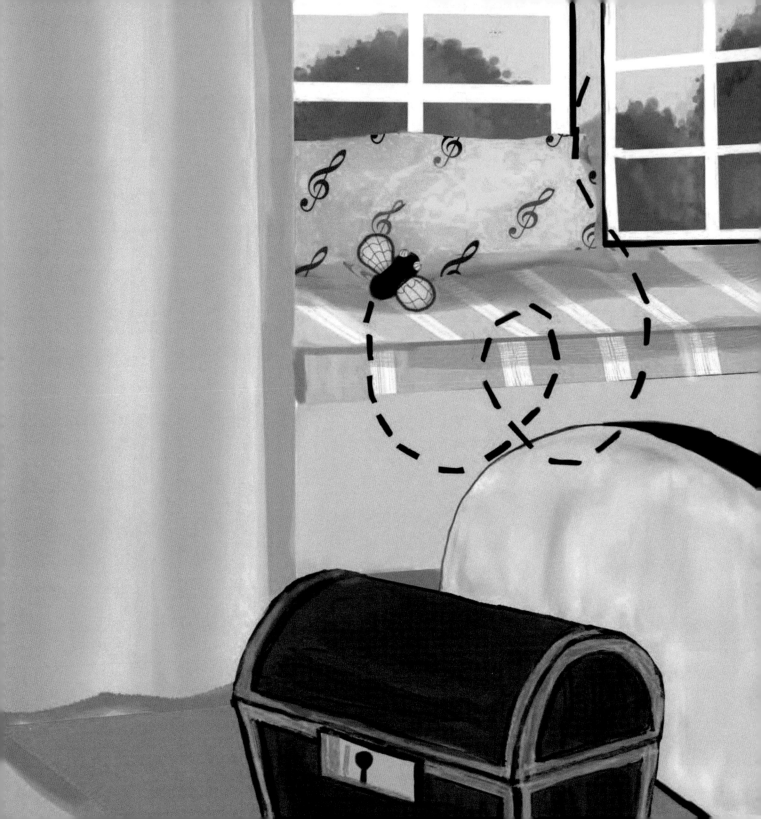

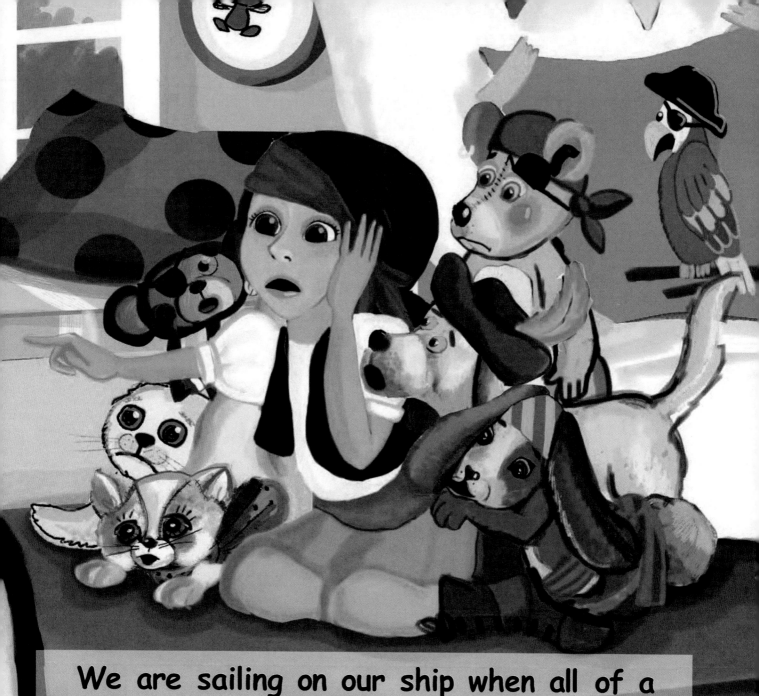

We are sailing on our ship when all of a sudden, a bug flies into my room. I scream and run out of my room! I do not like bugs!

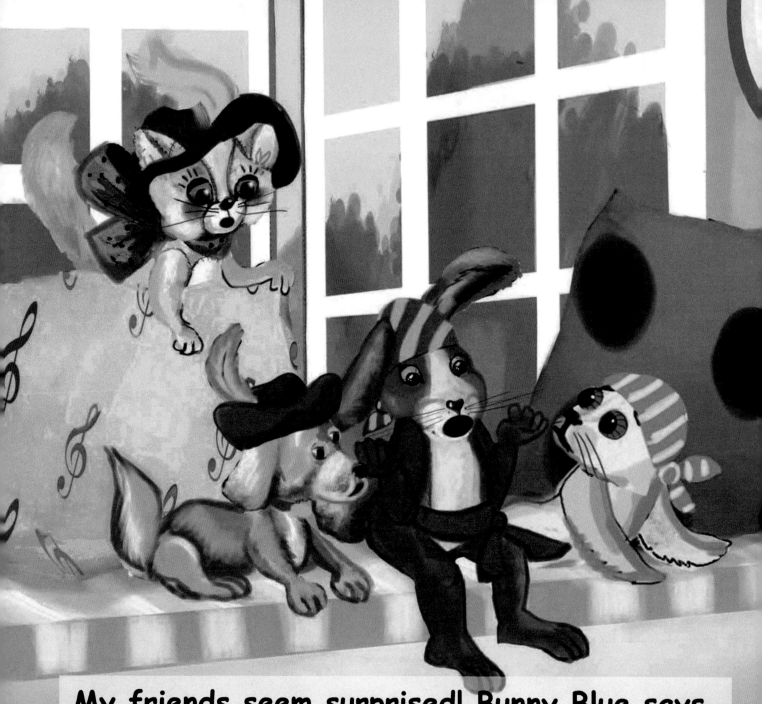

My friends seem surprised! Bunny Blue says,
"It is only a fly!"

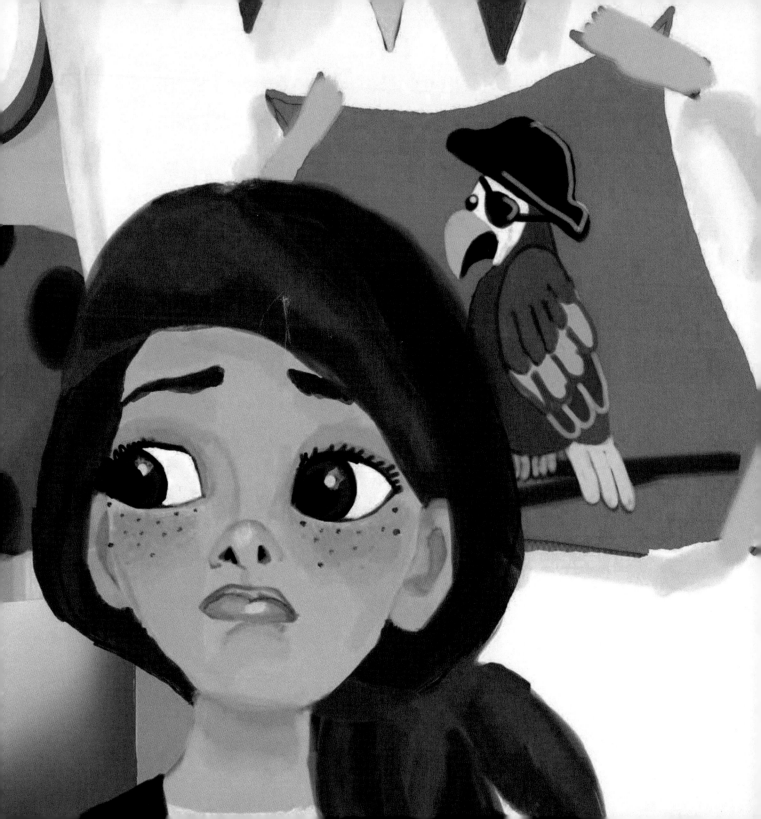

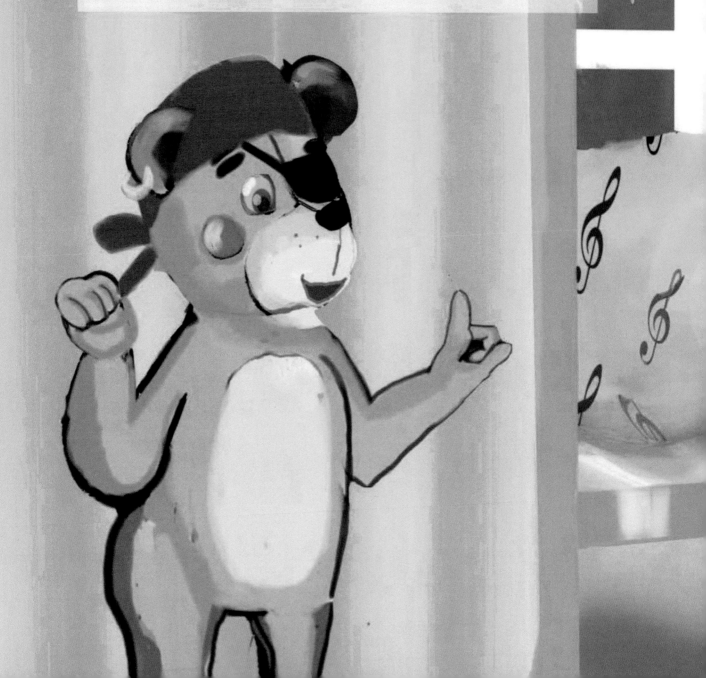

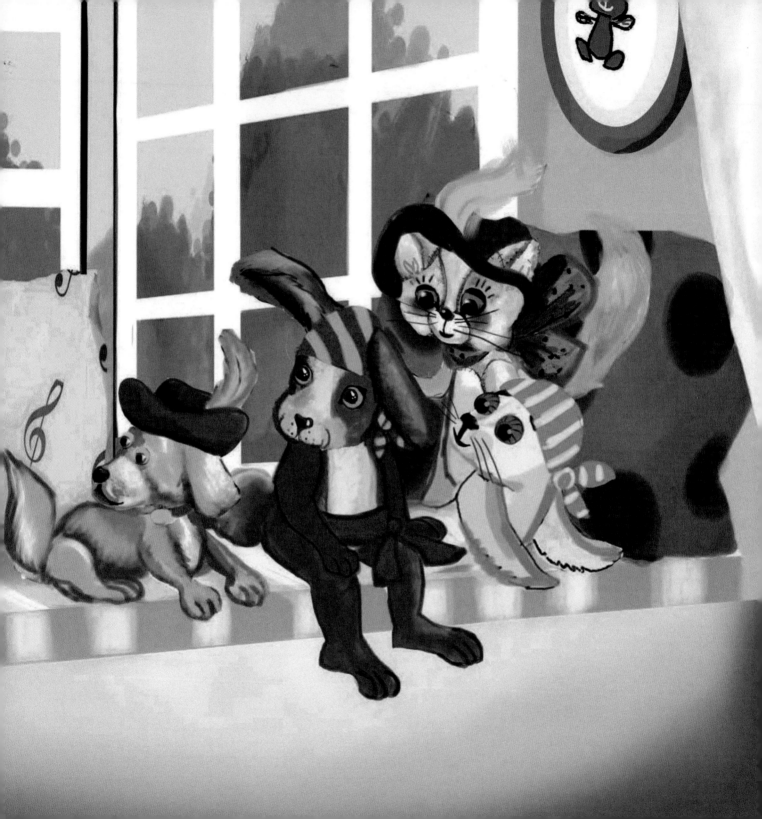

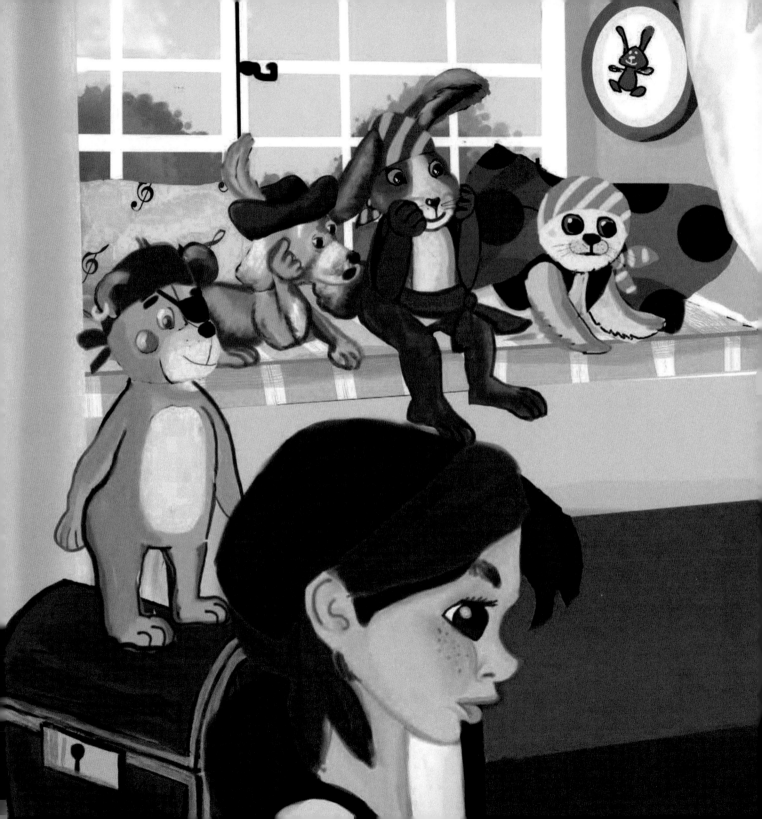

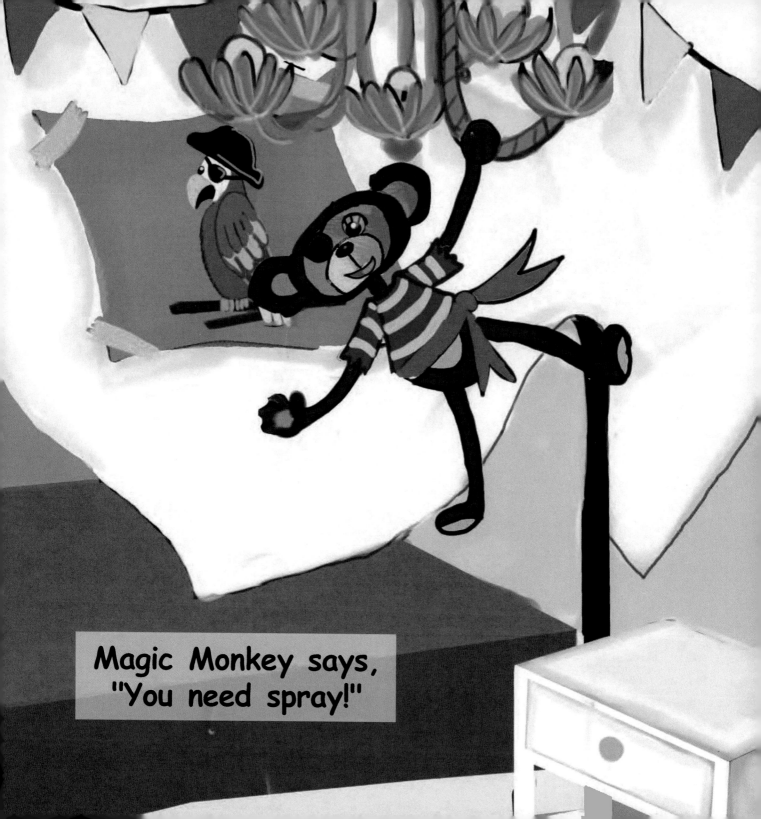

Magic Monkey says,
"You need spray!"

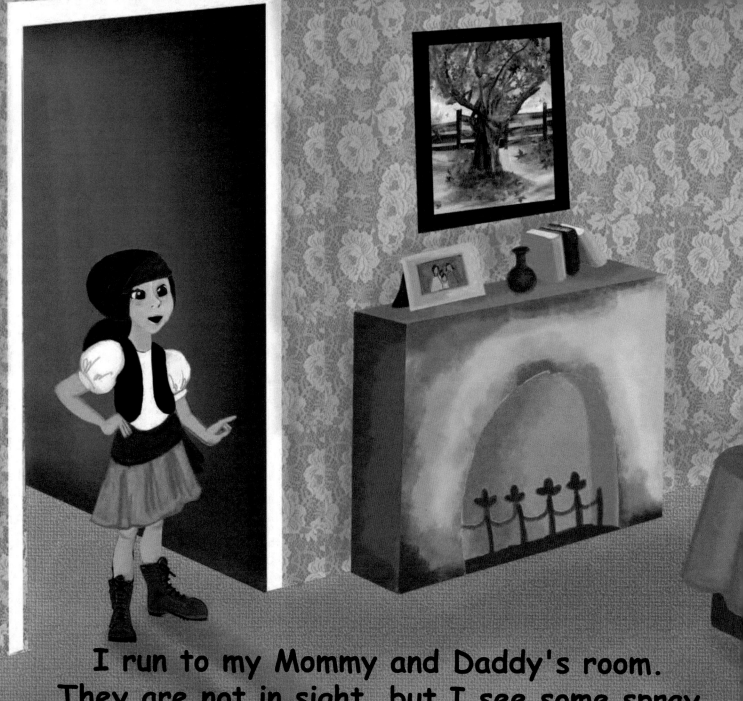

I run to my Mommy and Daddy's room.
They are not in sight, but I see some spray
on the dressing table. I quickly grab it and
run back to my room.

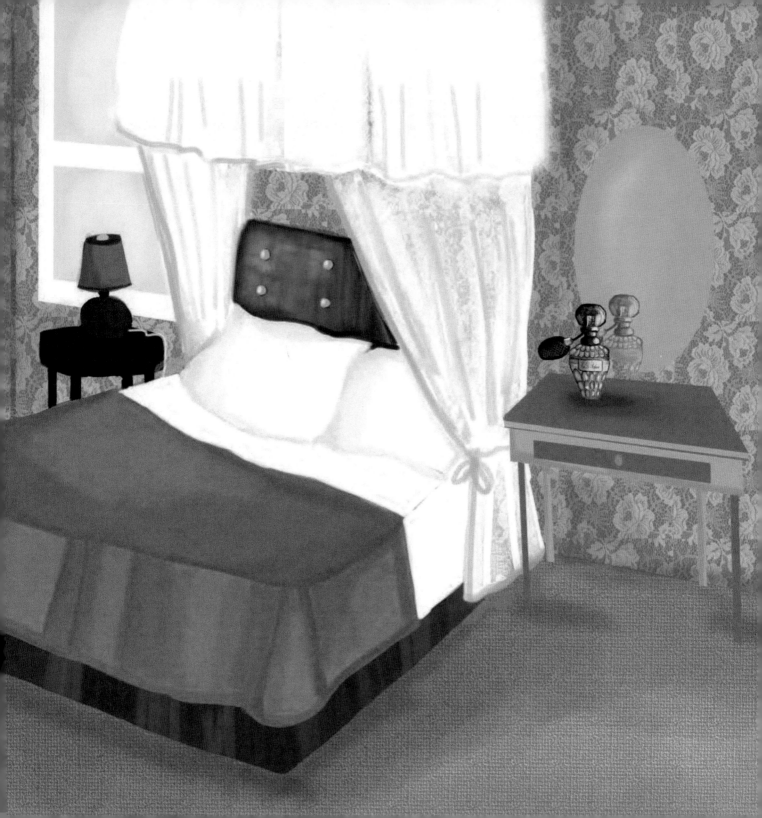

At first, I do not see the fly. Then playful Puppy says, "He is on my tail!" I spray his tail, but fly flies away.

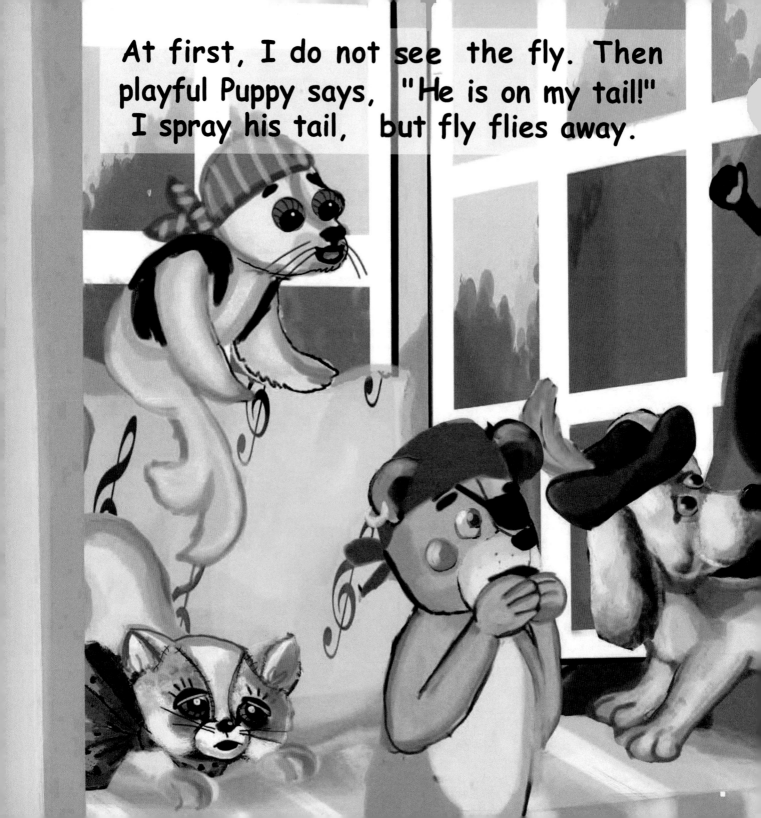

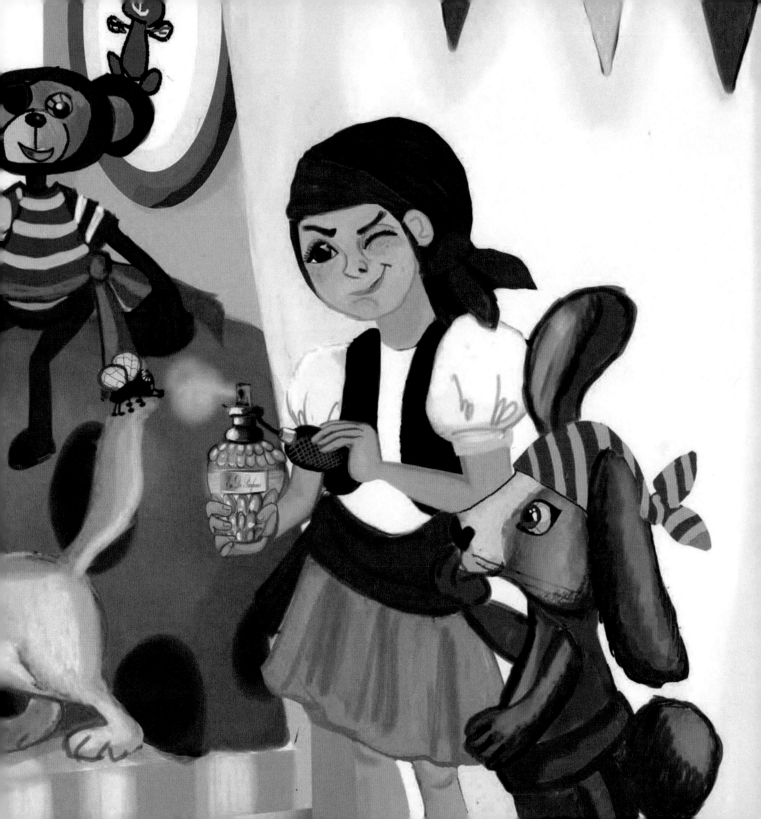

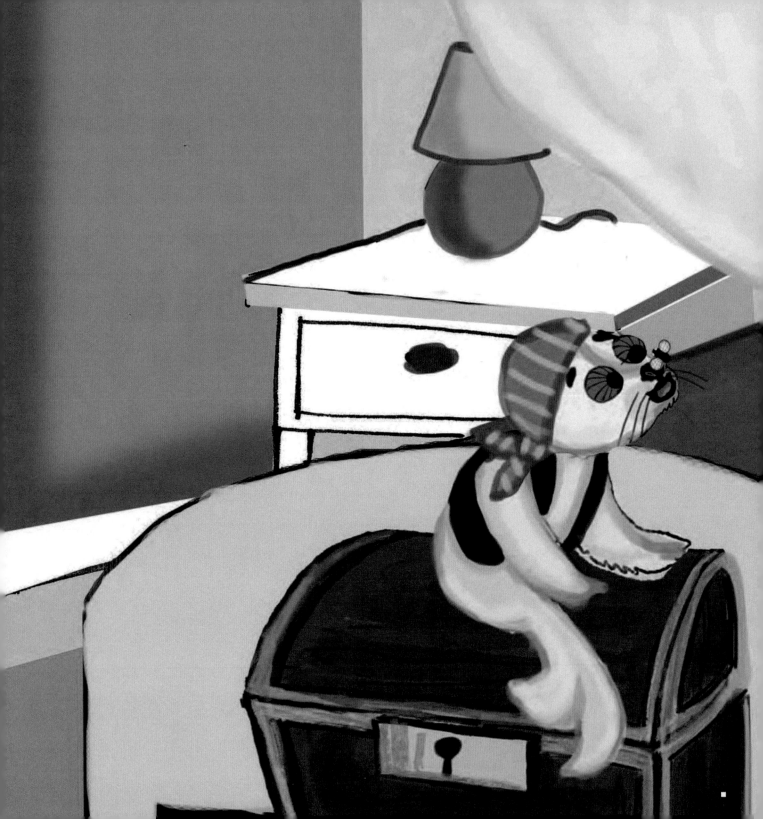

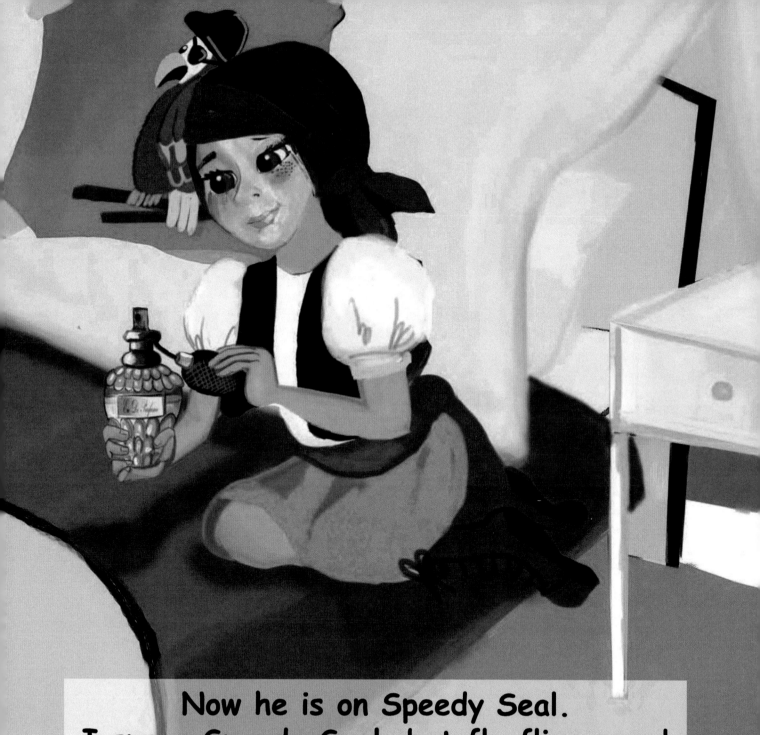

Now he is on Speedy Seal.
I spray Speedy Seal, but fly flies away!

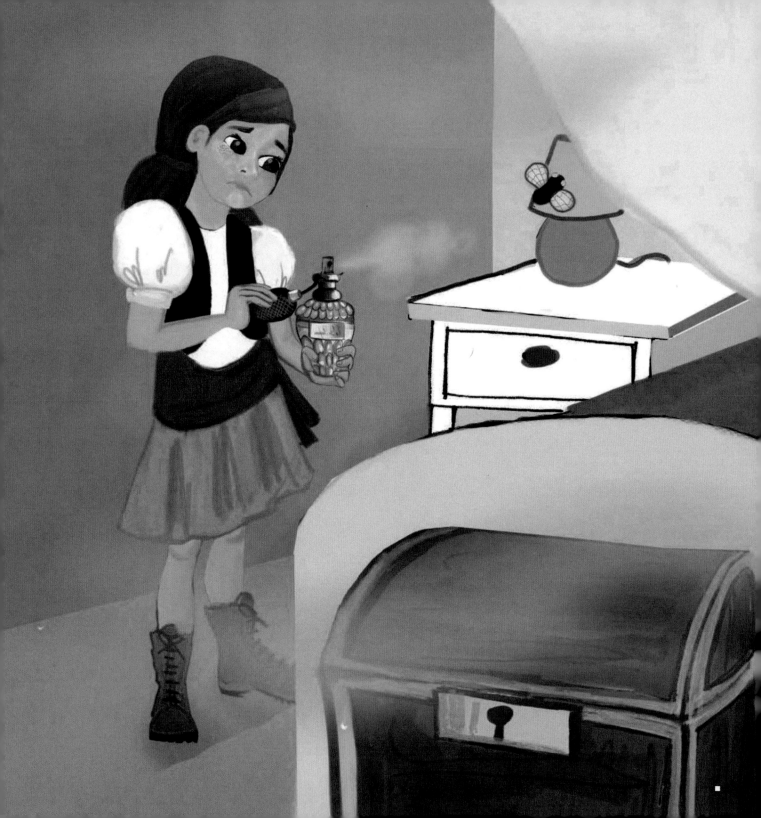

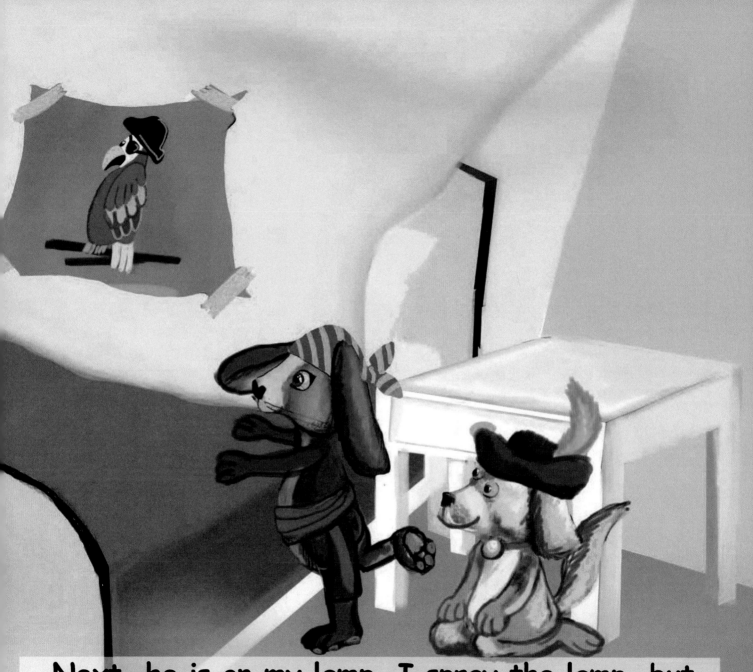

Next, he is on my lamp. I spray the lamp, but fly flies away. I spray here. I spray there. I spray everywhere. Fly keeps flying away!

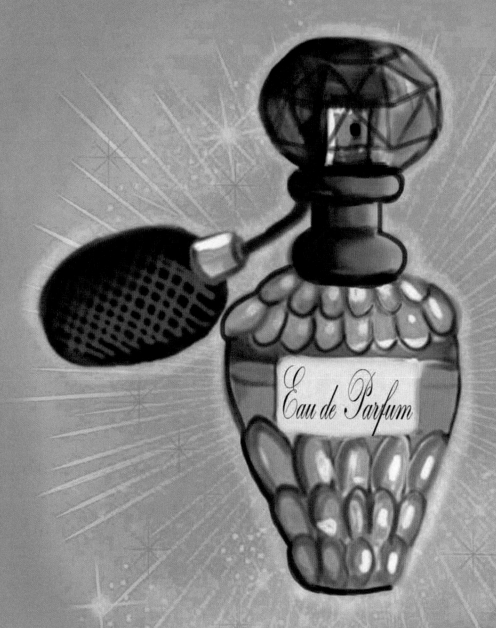

I notice my room smells very nice. I look at the spray. It is almost empty. I do not know the words on the spray.

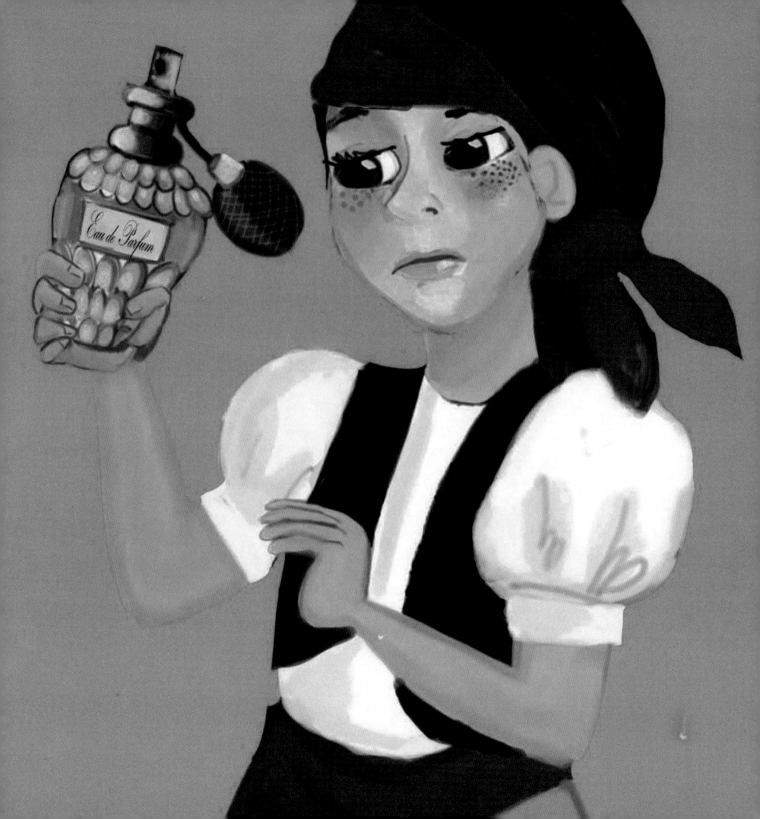

The label on the bottle reads: *Eau de Parfum*

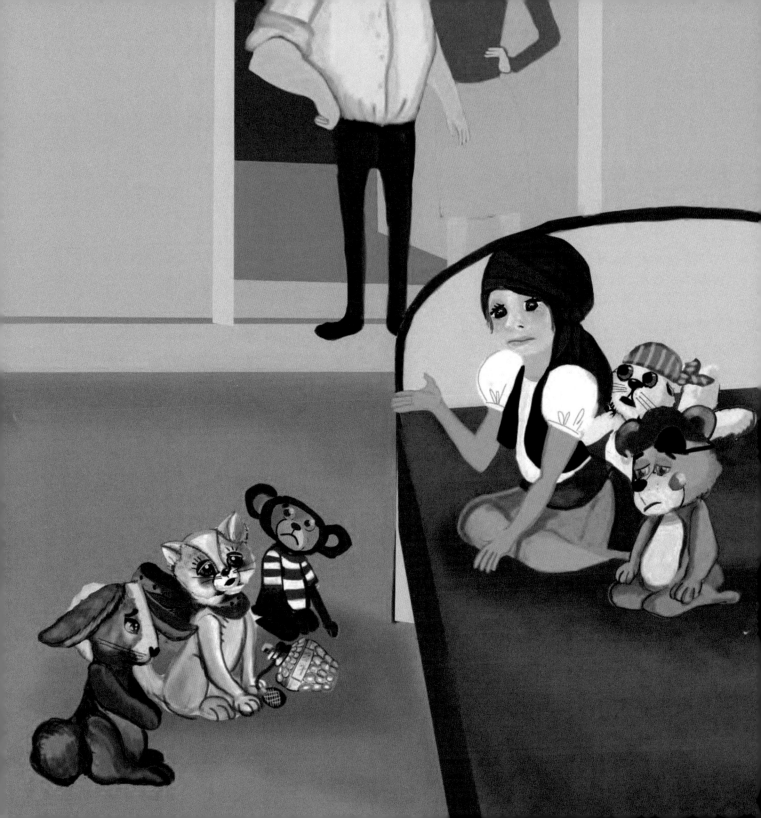

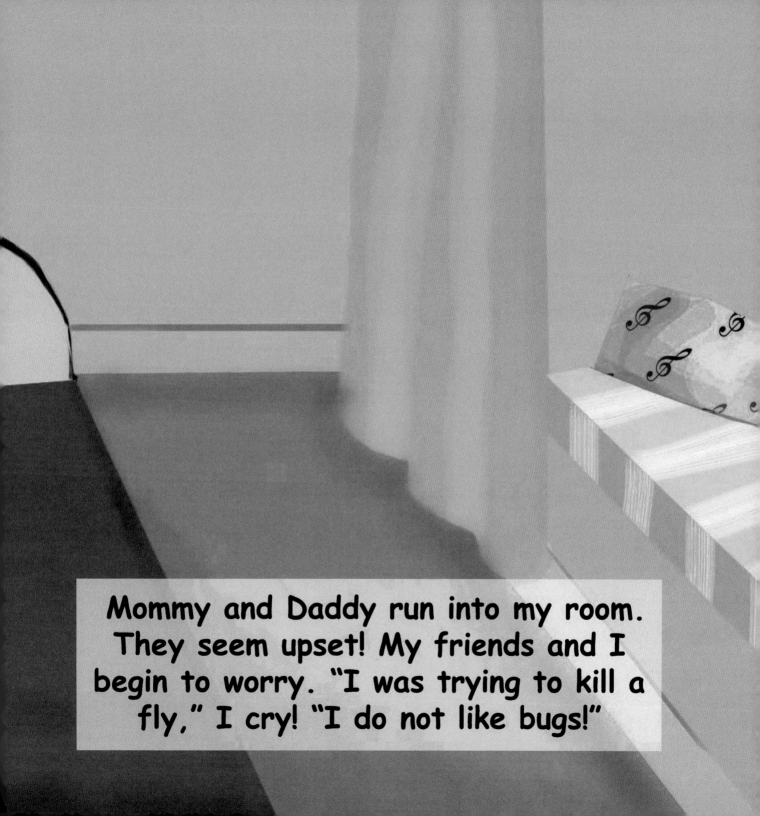

Mommy and Daddy run into my room. They seem upset! My friends and I begin to worry. "I was trying to kill a fly," I cry! "I do not like bugs!"

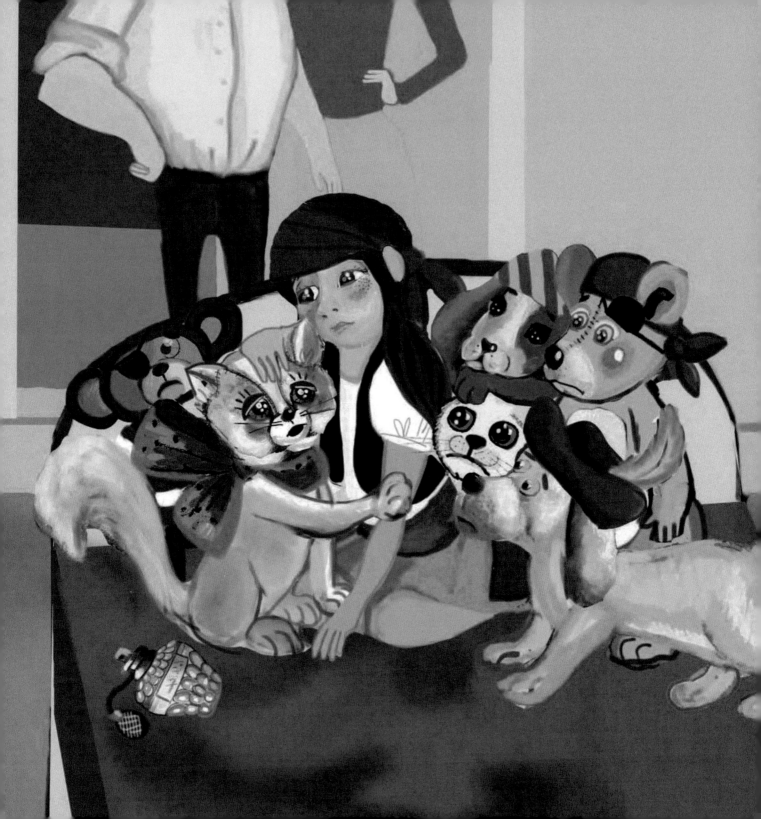

Daddy says, "Maybe you should ask for help." Just as he is saying this, the fly lands on my bed. I get scared! I do not like bugs! Then my Daddy says, "Oh look! There is Bob!"

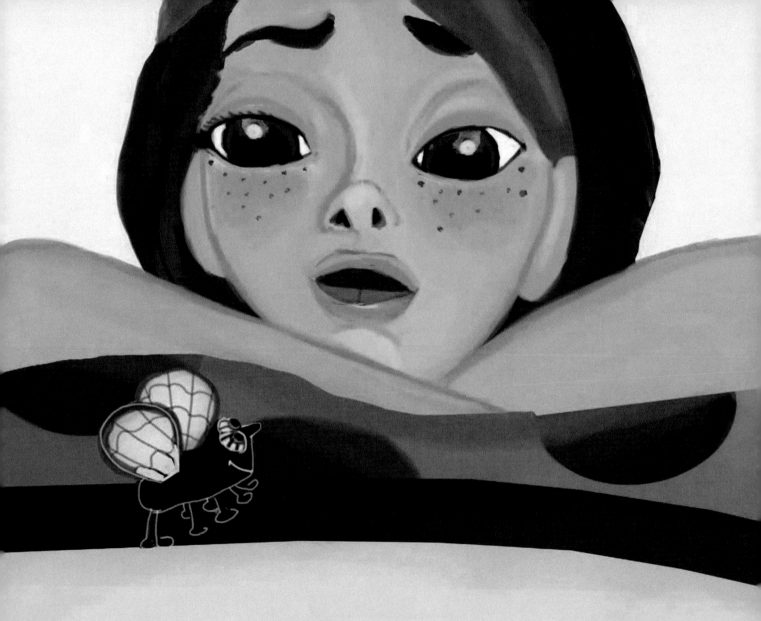

I look at the fly. The fly has a name?
The fly's name is Bob? I do not like
bugs, but this bug is Bob!

Daddy says,
"Would you like to get the fly swatter?"
I think about this for a minute. Bob does
not seem scary anymore!

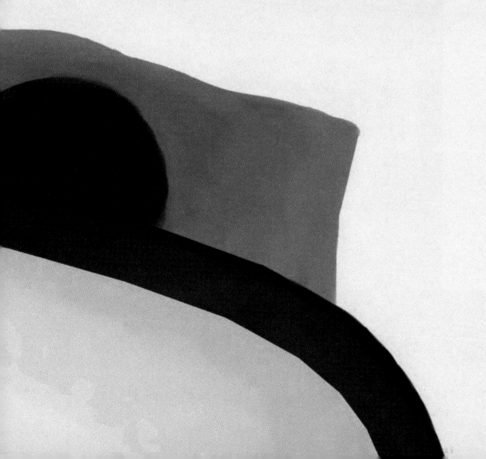

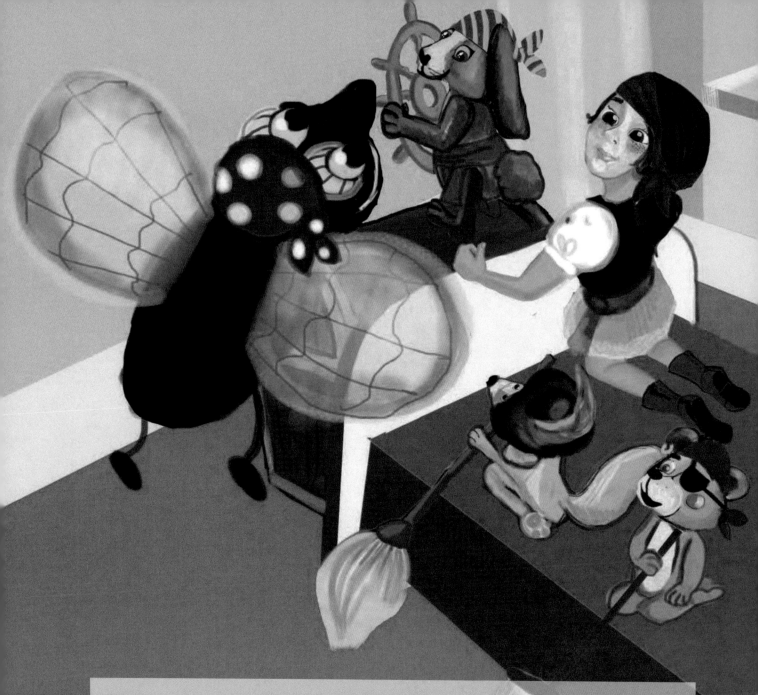

"No, it is okay. We are playing pirates.
I think Bob will be a dragon!"

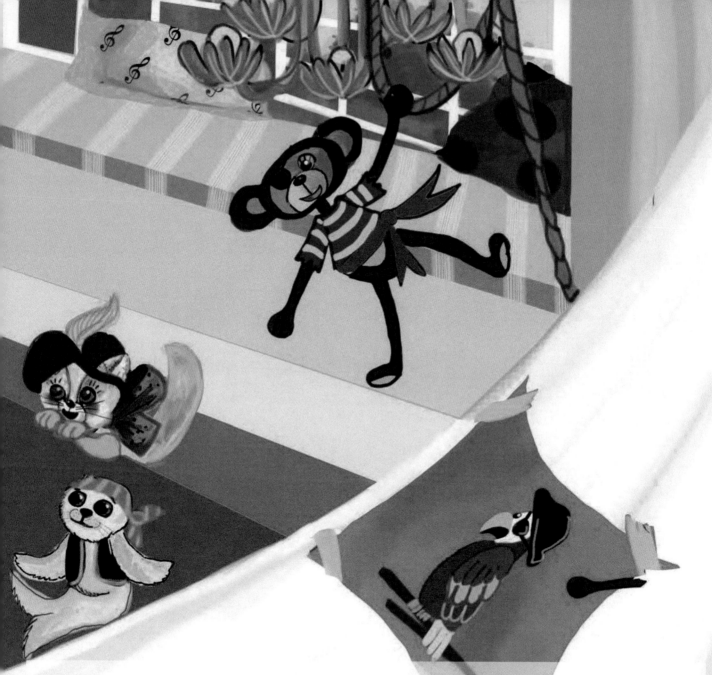

The pirate crew and I jump back on the ship.
The sea air smells sweet! Bob, the dragon,
flies overhead. It is a good day at sea!

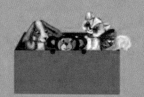
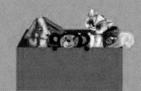
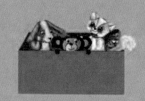

*I hope that reading
"I Do Not Like Bugs!"
was enjoyable for you and your child.
If so, please post a comment
on the books page on amazon.com.*

Thank you! P.T.

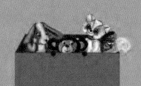
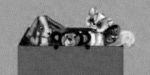

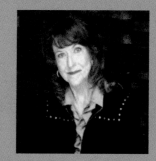

About the Author :

Pamela is the Author of children's books like a box of chocolates. Each book is sweet and unique. She wrote her first poem at the age of ten and has been writing ever since then. Above all else, she enjoys spending time with family and friends. She writes in the hope that it may somehow lift a burden and/or bring a smile to her readers. In the "My Truly Most Favorite Fluffy Friend" series, Emma and her friends help us under-stand the importance of values.

www.pamelatomlin.com

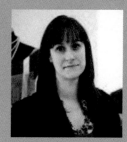

A Word from an Illustrator :

" As an artist from one small country named Serbia, it is a great honor to have worked with P. T. on this series. I devote every day of my life to my family and my art, and I hope I have been able to capture all the magic of Pamela's words with my illustrations."

pipertamr@gmail.com

Made in the USA
Coppell, TX
26 June 2020

29466007R00021